SCID-5-AMPD

STRUCTURED CLINICAL INTERVIEW FOR THE DSM-5® ALTERNATIVE MODEL FOR PERSONALITY DISORDERS

MODULE II

Structured Clinical Interview for **PERSONALITY TRAITS**

Andrew E. Skodol, M.D. • Michael B. First, M.D.
Donna S. Bender, Ph.D. • John M. Oldham, M.D.

Interviewee/ID#: _____   Interview date: _____ _____ _____
                                                              month   day   year

Clinician: _____

SCID-5-AMPD

STRUCTURED CLINICAL INTERVIEW FOR THE DSM-5®
ALTERNATIVE MODEL FOR PERSONALITY DISORDERS

MODULE II

STRUCTURED CLINICAL INTERVIEW FOR
PERSONALITY TRAITS

Andrew E. Skodol, M.D.
Research Professor of Psychiatry, University of Arizona College of Medicine,
Tucson, Arizona; and Adjunct Professor of Psychiatry, Columbia University College of
Physicians and Surgeons, New York, New York

Michael B. First, M.D.
Professor of Clinical Psychiatry, Columbia University College of Physicians and
Surgeons, and Research Psychiatrist, Division of Clinical Phenomenology,
New York State Psychiatric Institute, New York, New York

Donna S. Bender, Ph.D.
Director, Counseling and Psychological Services, and
Clinical Professor of Psychiatry and Behavioral Sciences,
Tulane University, New Orleans, Louisiana

John M. Oldham, M.D.
Professor of Psychiatry,
Barbara and Corbin Robertson Jr. Endowed Chair for Personality Disorders,
Baylor College of Medicine, Houston, Texas

An overview of the Module II rationale, structure, and approach is presented in the
User's Guide for the SCID-5-AMPD. Please refer to that manual for proper procedure
for conducting the assessment.

Contents

GENERAL OVERVIEW FOR THE SCID-5-AMPD

I'm going to start by asking you some questions about yourself and about problems or difficulties you may have had. I'll be making some notes as we go along. Do you have any questions before we begin?

NOTE: Any current suicidal thoughts, plans, or actions should be thoroughly assessed by the clinician and action taken if necessary.

DEMOGRAPHIC DATA

How old are you?

GENDER: ___ Male ___ Female ___ Other (e.g., transgender)

Are you married?

⟶ *IF YES:* **How long have you been married?**

⟶ *IF NO:* **Do you have a partner?**

    ⟶ *IF YES:* **How long have you been together? Do you live with your partner? Have you ever been married?**

    ⟶ *IF NO:* **Have you ever been married?**

IF EVER MARRIED: **How many times have you been married?**

Do you have any children?

    IF YES: **How many? (What are their ages?)**

With whom do you live? (How many children under the age of 18 live in your household?)

EDUCATION AND WORK HISTORY

How far did you go in school?

IF FAILED TO COMPLETE A PROGRAM IN WHICH INDIVIDUAL WAS ENROLLED:
Why did you leave?

What kind of work do you do? (Do you work outside of your home?)

Have you always done that kind of work?

    IF NO: **What other kind of work have you done in the past?**

What's the longest you've worked at one place?

(continued on next page)

EDUCATION AND WORK HISTORY (*continued*)

Are you currently employed (getting paid)?

IF NO: **Why not?**

IF UNKNOWN: **Has there ever been a period of time when you were unable to work or go to school?**

IF YES: **Why was that?**

Have you ever been arrested, involved in a lawsuit, or had other legal trouble?

CURRENT AND PAST PERIODS OF PSYCHOPATHOLOGY

Have you ever seen anybody for emotional or psychiatric problems?

IF YES: **What was that for? (What treatment did you get? Any medications? When was that? When was the first time you ever saw someone for emotional or psychiatric problems?)**

IF NO: **Was there ever a time when you, or someone else, thought you should see someone because of the way you were feeling or acting? (Tell me more.)**

Have you ever seen anybody for problems with alcohol or drugs?

IF YES: **What was that for? (What treatment[s] did you get? Any medications? When was that?)**

Have you ever attended a self-help group, like Alcoholics Anonymous, Gamblers Anonymous, or Overeaters Anonymous?

IF YES: **What was that for? When was that?**

Thinking back over your whole life, have there been times when things were not going well for you or when you were emotionally upset? (Tell me about that. When was that? What was that like? What was going on? How were you feeling?)

INTERVIEWER INSTRUCTIONS

In the Alternative Model, personality traits, also known as "facets," are grouped into five broad trait domains: Negative Affectivity, Detachment, Antagonism, Disinhibition, and Psychoticism. A *personality trait* is a tendency to feel, perceive, behave, and think in relatively consistent ways across time and across situations in which the trait may be manifested. **Ask all of the questions for each facet and then make a single, overall rating of the degree to which each facet describes the interviewee.** For each question, ask for examples and elaboration until you have sufficient information to make a judgment. You should ensure that elicited examples represent actual traits (i.e., general predispositions or tendencies) as opposed to more limited instances of behavior. **In some cases to minimize redundancy, it may make sense to skip a question in the assessment of a facet if the answer is already clear from previous information.**

There are four columns in this interview schedule:

1. The left-hand column contains the interview questions.
2. The second column shows the facet name and its domain.
3. The third column contains the definition of the facet.
4. The fourth, right-most column is used to record the trait ratings.

Personality facets within each domain are rated on a four-point scale of descriptiveness: **0 = "Very little or not at all descriptive," 1 = "Mildly descriptive," 2 = "Moderately descriptive," 3 = "Very descriptive."** The facets should describe the interviewee's current personality and be descriptive for at least the past 2 years. The facet descriptions usually contain multiple components (e.g., the Impulsivity facet in Borderline and Antisocial Personality Disorders includes three components: "acting on the spur of the moment in response to immediate stimuli," "acting on a momentary basis without a plan or consideration of outcomes," and "difficulty establishing and following plans"). **A rating of "3" does not necessarily require that all of the components are descriptive of the individual. If some subset of components is particularly descriptive, a rating of "3" may still be appropriate.** For example, an individual may be very prone to acting on the spur of the moment without considering the outcomes but still be able to establish or follow a plan. **A rating of "?" indicates that there is insufficient information to make a judgment about the descriptiveness of the facet.**

At the end of each domain section, the interviewer records the scores for the individual trait facets in that domain and calculates a total score and an average score for the domain in the space provided. To enhance the flow of the interview, the domain scoring can be skipped until all the interview questions have been asked and the interview completed. The interviewer can then tally the scores separately. These scores are then transferred to page 33 of the interview to provide a profile of the interviewee's personality in terms of domains and a summary of average scores.

Begin Module II with the following questions to get a basic sense of the interviewee's characteristic personality style with respect to emotional life, affiliations with and attitudes toward others, impulse control, thinking, and perception.

PRELIMINARY QUESTIONS ABOUT VIEW OF SELF AND QUALITY OF INTERPERSONAL RELATIONSHIPS

IF THE QUESTIONS BELOW HAVE ALREADY BEEN ASKED IN THE CONTEXT OF ADMINISTERING MODULE I, SKIP THIS SECTION AND PROCEED WITH THE EVALUATION OF **NEGATIVE AFFECTIVITY DOMAIN**, *PAGE 6.*

The purpose of this interview is to explore different ways in which you see yourself, your basic approach to life, and how you interact with other people. Let's start with some general questions about how you are as a person:

1.   **How would you describe yourself as a person?**

2.   **How do you think other people describe you?**

3.   **How do you generally feel about yourself?**

(continued on next page)

4.   How successful would you say you are at getting the things you want in life?
       (Like having a satisfying relationship, a fulfilling career, close friends?)

5.   What are your relationships with other people like?

6.   Who are the most important people in your life? How do you get along with them?

7.   How well do you think you understand yourself?

8.   How well do you understand other people?

NEGATIVE AFFECTIVITY DOMAIN

Frequent and intense experiences of high levels of a wide range of negative emotions
(e.g., anxiety, depression, guilt/shame, worry, anger) and their behavioral (e.g., self-harm)
and interpersonal (e.g., dependency) manifestations.

Interview questions	Facets	General definition	Trait ratings
	Emotional Lability (an aspect of Negative Affectivity)		? 0 1 2 3
Would you consider yourself to be a very emotional person? *IF NO:* **Do other people consider you to be very moody?**		Instability of emotional experiences and mood;	
Do your emotions often change suddenly, quickly going from happy to angry or sad?		Emotions that are easily aroused, intense, and/or out of proportion to events and circumstances.	
Do you tend to react very strongly to things that happen to you? *IF NO:* **Have people told you that your emotional reactions are more intense than they should be, given the circumstances?**			

?	0	1	2	3
Insufficient information	**Very little or not at all descriptive**	**Mildly descriptive**	**Moderately descriptive**	**Very descriptive**

Interview questions	Facets	General definition	Trait ratings
	Anxiousness (an aspect of Negative Affectivity)		? 0 1 2 3
Do you generally feel very nervous, anxious, or even panicky in a variety of situations?		Feelings of nervousness, tenseness, or panic in reaction to diverse situations;	
Are you almost always worrying about something?			
Do you tend to dwell on the bad things that have happened to you in the past?		Frequent worry about the negative effects of past unpleasant experiences and future negative possibilities;	
What about worrying about bad things that might happen to you in the future?			
Do you tend to feel upset when things are up in the air or when you are uncertain about how things will turn out?		Feeling fearful and apprehensive about uncertainty; expecting the worst to happen.	
Do you almost always expect the worst will happen to you and other people you care about?			

?	0	1	2	3
Insufficient information	Very little or not at all descriptive	Mildly descriptive	Moderately descriptive	Very descriptive

Interview questions	Facets	General definition	Trait ratings
Do you often worry that you will be rejected or abandoned by people you are involved with? Do you tend to get very anxious when you are separated from those you depend on? Do you worry a lot about being left alone to take care of yourself physically or emotionally?	**Separation Insecurity** (an aspect of Negative Affectivity)	Fears of being alone due to rejection by—and/or separation from—significant others, based in a lack of confidence in one's ability to care for oneself, both physically and emotionally.	? 0 1 2 3
Do you find it hard to disagree with people even when you think they are wrong? Do you tend to put other people's interests, needs, or desires before your own even when they go against your own? Do you always try to find out what other people want before deciding what you want for yourself? Do you usually do what you think others want you to do?	**Submissiveness** (an aspect of Negative Affectivity)	Adaptation of one's behavior to the actual or perceived interests and desires of others even when doing so is antithetical to one's own interests, needs, or desires.	? 0 1 2 3

?	0	1	2	3
Insufficient information	Very little or not at all descriptive	Mildly descriptive	Moderately descriptive	Very descriptive

Interview questions	Facets	General definition	Trait ratings
	Hostility (an aspect of Negative Affectivity and Antagonism)		? 0 1 2 3
Are you angry much of the time?		Persistent or frequent angry feelings;	
Are you easily angered?			
Do you often get angry or lash out when someone criticizes or insults you in some way?		Anger or irritability in response to minor slights and insults;	
Do you often snap at people when they do little things that irritate you?			
Do you feel it's very important to get back at people who have hurt you or done you wrong?		Mean, nasty, or vengeful behavior.	
Would you say that you have a mean or nasty streak?			

?	0	1	2	3
Insufficient information	Very little or not at all descriptive	Mildly descriptive	Moderately descriptive	Very descriptive

Interview questions	Facets	General definition	Trait ratings
	Perseveration (an aspect of Negative Affectivity)		? 0 1 2 3
Do you tend to keep doing the same thing over and over again even though it is not getting you anywhere?		Persistence at tasks or in a particular way of doing things long after the behavior has ceased to be functional or effective;	
Do you tend to keep doing certain things the same way, even when it's clear that your approach is not working?		Continuance of the same behavior despite repeated failures or clear reasons for stopping. *[Note: Addictive behaviors such as substance use or gambling and compulsive self-injurious behaviors should not be considered as evidence for this trait.]*	

?	0	1	2	3
Insufficient information	**Very little or not at all descriptive**	**Mildly descriptive**	**Moderately descriptive**	**Very descriptive**

Negative Affectivity Domain Score

Record each <u>Negative Affectivity facet</u> score here:

Emotional Lability	_____
Anxiousness	_____
Separation Insecurity	_____
Submissiveness	_____
Hostility	_____
Perseveration	_____
Depressivity (rating obtained in Detachment Domain, page 14)	_____
Suspiciousness (rating obtained in Detachment Domain, page 16)	_____
Sum of the above scores (record on page 33, "Personality Trait Domain Profile")	_____
Average score (summed scores divided by 8) (record on page 33, "Summary of Average Domain Scores")	_____

?	0	1	2	3
Insufficient information	**Very little or not at all descriptive**	**Mildly descriptive**	**Moderately descriptive**	**Very descriptive**

DETACHMENT DOMAIN

Avoidance of socioemotional experience, including both withdrawal from interpersonal interactions (ranging from casual, daily interactions to friendships to intimate relationships) and restricted affective experience and expression, particularly limited hedonic capacity.

Interview questions	Facets	General definition	Trait ratings
	Withdrawal (an aspect of Detachment)		? 0 1 2 3
Would you almost always rather do things alone than with other people? Why is that?		Preference for being alone to being with others;	
Are you usually quiet when you meet new people?		Reticence in social situations;	
Do you generally try to avoid social events?		Avoidance of social contacts and activity;	
Do you usually avoid starting conversations with people you don't know very well?		Lack of initiation of social contact.	

?	0	1	2	3
Insufficient information	**Very little or not at all descriptive**	**Mildly descriptive**	**Moderately descriptive**	**Very descriptive**

Interview questions	Facets	General definition	Trait ratings
IF UNKNOWN: **What's the most satisfying romantic or sexual relationship that you have had? Tell me about it.** *ASK THE FOLLOWING QUESTIONS ONLY IF UNCLEAR FROM RELATIONSHIP HISTORY:* **Do you tend to avoid getting close to people? Why is that?** **Do you tend to break off relationships or friendships if they start to get close?** **Have you generally avoided getting into emotionally intimate sexual relationships?**	**Intimacy Avoidance** (an aspect of Detachment)	Avoidance of close or romantic relationships, interpersonal attachments, and intimate sexual relationships.	? 0 1 2 3
Are there really very few things that give you pleasure? **Do you feel like you don't have enough energy to take advantage of what life has to offer?** **Do you find that you do not get as much pleasure out of things as others seem to?** **Do you find that nothing seems to interest you very much?**	**Anhedonia** (an aspect of Detachment)	Lack of enjoyment from, engagement in, or energy for life's experiences; Deficits in the capacity to feel pleasure and take interest in things.	? 0 1 2 3

?	0	1	2	3
Insufficient information	Very little or not at all descriptive	Mildly descriptive	Moderately descriptive	Very descriptive

Interview questions	Facets	General definition	Trait ratings
	Depressivity (an aspect of Negative Affectivity and Detachment)		? 0 1 2 3
Do you often feel down, depressed, or miserable?		Feelings of being down, miserable, and/or hopeless;	
Does the future look really hopeless to you?			
Once you start feeling depressed, is it hard for you to snap out of it?		Difficulty recovering from such moods;	
Do you almost always expect things to turn out badly?		Pessimism about the future;	
Do you feel ashamed about a lot of things? What about?		Pervasive shame and/or guilt;	
Do you feel guilty much of the time about things you have done or not done? What about?			
Do you believe that you are basically an inadequate person and often don't feel good about yourself?		Feelings of inferior self-worth;	
Do you often feel like a failure?			
	(*continued on next page*)		

?	0	1	2	3
Insufficient information	**Very little or not at all descriptive**	**Mildly descriptive**	**Moderately descriptive**	**Very descriptive**

Interview questions	Facets	General definition	Trait ratings
	Depressivity (*continued*)		
Do you generally feel like the world would be better off if you were dead?		Thoughts of suicide and suicidal behavior.	
Have you sometimes had thoughts of killing yourself?			
Have you ever done anything to try to take your own life or made plans to do so?			
	Restricted Affectivity (an aspect of Detachment)		? 0 1 2 3
Do you tend not to get emotional about things?		Little reaction to emotionally arousing situations;	
Do you find that books, movies, and music that other people find moving leave you cold?			
Do you find that nothing makes you very happy or very sad or very angry?		Constricted emotional experience and expression;	
Have people told you that it is difficult to know what you're feeling?			
Do you not seem to care about anything or anyone?		Indifference and aloofness in normatively engaging situations.	
IF NO: **Have other people complained that you are an indifferent or aloof person?**			

?	0	1	2	3
Insufficient information	Very little or not at all descriptive	Mildly descriptive	Moderately descriptive	Very descriptive

Interview questions	Facets	General definition	Trait ratings
	Suspiciousness (an aspect of Negative Affectivity and Detachment)		? 0 1 2 3
Do you often have to keep an eye out to stop people from using you or hurting you?		Expectations of—and sensitivity to—signs of interpersonal ill-intent or harm;	
Are you especially sensitive to how other people treat you?			
Do you find that it is best not to let other people know much about you because they will use it against you?			
Have you often suspected that your spouse or partner has been unfaithful?		Doubts about loyalty and fidelity of others;	
Do you spend a lot of time wondering if you can trust your friends or the people you work with?		Feelings of being mistreated, used, and/or persecuted by others.	
Do you often feel like you are being harassed or treated cruelly or unfairly by others?			

?	0	1	2	3
Insufficient information	Very little or not at all descriptive	Mildly descriptive	Moderately descriptive	Very descriptive

Detachment Domain Score

Record each <u>Detachment facet</u> score here:

Withdrawal	_____
Intimacy Avoidance	_____
Anhedonia	_____
Depressivity	_____
Restricted Affectivity	_____
Suspiciousness	_____
Sum of the above scores (record on page 33, "Personality Trait Domain Profile")	_____
Average score (summed scores divided by 6) (record on page 33, "Summary of Average Domain Scores")	_____

?	**0**	**1**	**2**	**3**
Insufficient information	Very little or not at all descriptive	Mildly descriptive	Moderately descriptive	Very descriptive

ANTAGONISM DOMAIN

Behaviors that put the individual at odds with other people, including an exaggerated
sense of self-importance and a concomitant expectation of special treatment,
as well as a callous antipathy toward others, encompassing both an unawareness of others' needs
and feelings and a readiness to use others in the service of self-enhancement.

Interview questions	Facets	General definition	Trait ratings
	Manipulativeness (an aspect of Antagonism)		?　0　1　2　3
Are you good at making other people do what you want them to?		Use of subterfuge to influence or control others;	
Is it easy for you to take advantage of others?			
Do you bend the truth in order to get other people to do what you need them to do?			
Do you often "turn on the charm" or behave seductively in order to get what you want?		Use of seduction, charm, glibness, or ingratiation to achieve one's ends.	
Do you praise people when you don't mean it in order to get them to do what you want?			

?	0	1	2	3
Insufficient information	Very little or not at all descriptive	Mildly descriptive	Moderately descriptive	Very descriptive

Interview questions	Facets	General definition	Trait ratings
	Deceitfulness (an aspect of Antagonism)		**? 0 1 2 3**
Do you tend to exaggerate in order to get ahead?		Dishonesty and fraudulence;	
Do you often cheat in order to get what you want?			
Do you find that lying comes easily to you?			
Have you often "conned" others to get what you want?			
Have you ever used an "alias" or pretended you were somebody else?		Misrepresentation of self;	
Do you tend to make things up when telling others about yourself?		Embellishment or fabrication when relating events.	
Do you often make up stories about things that happened that are totally untrue?			

?	0	1	2	3
Insufficient information	Very little or not at all descriptive	Mildly descriptive	Moderately descriptive	Very descriptive

Interview questions	Facets	General definition	Trait ratings
	Grandiosity (an aspect of Antagonism)		? 0 1 2 3
Do you feel like you have unique qualities that few others possess?		Believing that one is superior to others and deserves special treatment;	
Do you feel like you're more important than most people?			
Do you often feel resentful that other people fail to appreciate your special qualities or abilities?			
Have people told you that you have too high an opinion of yourself?			
Have other people told you that you are self-centered and only talk about yourself?		Self-centeredness;	
Do you think it's not necessary to follow certain rules or social conventions when they get in the way?		Feelings of entitlement;	
Do you feel that you are the kind of person who deserves special treatment?			
Do you find that there are very few people who are worth your time and attention?		Condescension toward others.	

?	0	1	2	3
Insufficient information	Very little or not at all descriptive	Mildly descriptive	Moderately descriptive	Very descriptive

Interview questions	Facets	General definition	Trait ratings
	Attention Seeking (an aspect of Antagonism)		? 0 1 2 3
Do you like to be the center of attention? Do you try to draw attention to yourself by the way you act, dress, or look? Do you often do things in order to get others to admire you? Do you like standing out in a crowd?		Engaging in behavior designed to attract notice and to make oneself the focus of others' attention and admiration.	
	Callousness (an aspect of Antagonism)		? 0 1 2 3
Do you tend to feel that other people's feelings or problems are not your concern? Do you generally feel like it's no big deal if you hurt other people's feelings? If someone gets hurt because of something you do, do you feel guilty or sorry?		Lack of concern for the feelings or problems of others; Lack of guilt or remorse about the negative or harmful effects of one's actions on others.	

? Insufficient information	0 Very little or not at all descriptive	1 Mildly descriptive	2 Moderately descriptive	3 Very descriptive

Antagonism Domain Score

Record each <u>Antagonism facet</u> score here:

Manipulativeness	_____
Deceitfulness	_____
Grandiosity	_____
Attention Seeking	_____
Callousness	_____
Hostility (rating obtained in Negative Affectivity Domain, page 9)	_____
Sum of the above scores (record on page 33, "Personality Trait Domain Profile")	_____
Average score (summed scores divided by 6) (record on page 33, "Summary of Average Domain Scores")	_____

?	**0**	**1**	**2**	**3**
Insufficient information	**Very little or not at all descriptive**	**Mildly descriptive**	**Moderately descriptive**	**Very descriptive**

DISINHIBITION DOMAIN

Orientation toward immediate gratification, leading to impulsive behavior driven by current thoughts, feelings, and external stimuli, without regard for past learning or consideration of future consequences.

Interview questions	Facets	General definition	Trait ratings
	Irresponsibility (an aspect of Disinhibition)		? 0 1 2 3
Have you ever owed people money and not paid them back?		Disregard for—and failure to honor—financial and other obligations or commitments;	
What about not paying child support or not giving money to children or someone else who depended on you?			
Have you ever filed for bankruptcy? (How many times?)			
Do you tend to make promises that you don't keep?		Lack of respect for—and lack of follow-through on—agreements and promises;	
Do you tend to skip important meetings and appointments if you don't feel like going?			
Do others consider you to be irresponsible?			
Have people not wanted to lend you things like tools, books, or clothing because you haven't returned them or returned them in bad condition?		Carelessness with others' property.	

?	0	1	2	3
Insufficient information	Very little or not at all descriptive	Mildly descriptive	Moderately descriptive	Very descriptive

Interview questions	Facets	General definition	Trait ratings
	Impulsivity (an aspect of Disinhibition)		? 0 1 2 3
Do you often do things on the spur of the moment without thinking about how it will affect you or other people?		Acting on the spur of the moment in response to immediate stimuli;	
When something happens to you, do you usually react immediately and without thinking about it? Tell me about that.			
Have you often done things impulsively, like buying things you really couldn't afford, having sex with people you hardly knew, having unsafe sex, or driving recklessly?		Acting on a momentary basis without a plan or consideration of outcomes;	
Do you find that you often make rash decisions without adequately considering the possible outcomes?			
Do you find it difficult to make plans or to stick with them?		Difficulty establishing and following plans;	
When you are under a lot of stress, do you do things such as cutting, burning, or scratching yourself?		A sense of urgency and self-harming behavior under emotional distress.	
IF YES: **Do you feel a sense of urgency to do these things?**			

?	0	1	2	3
Insufficient information	Very little or not at all descriptive	Mildly descriptive	Moderately descriptive	Very descriptive

Interview questions	Facets	General definition	Trait ratings
	Distractibility (an aspect of Disinhibition)		? 0 1 2 3
Do you tend to find it hard to concentrate and focus on tasks?		Difficulty concentrating and focusing on tasks; attention is easily diverted by extraneous stimuli;	
Do you tend to be easily distracted by things around you so that you have trouble concentrating or staying on one track?			
Do you have trouble pursuing specific goals, even for short periods of time?		Difficulty maintaining goal-focused behavior, including both planning and completing tasks.	
Do you have trouble planning and completing tasks?			
	Risk Taking (an aspect of Disinhibition)		? 0 1 2 3
Are you drawn to thrilling activities, even if they are very dangerous or risky?		Engagement in dangerous, risky, and potentially self-damaging activities, unnecessarily and without regard to consequences;	
Do you often engage in dangerous or risky activities regardless of your lack of training or experience?		Lack of concern for one's limitations and denial of the reality of personal danger;	
Would other people describe you as reckless?		Reckless pursuit of goals regardless of the level of risk involved.	
Do you do a lot of things that others would consider risky?			

?	0	1	2	3
Insufficient information	Very little or not at all descriptive	Mildly descriptive	Moderately descriptive	Very descriptive

Interview questions	Facets	General definition	Trait ratings
	Rigid Perfectionism (an aspect of extreme Conscientiousness, the opposite of Disinhibition)		? 0 1 2 3
Do you insist on perfection in everything you do? Tell me about that.		Rigid insistence on everything being flawless, perfect, and without errors or faults, including one's own and others' performance;	
Do you also insist that everything other people do be flawless and perfect?			
Do you have trouble finishing jobs because you spend so much time trying to get things exactly right?		Sacrificing of timeliness to ensure correctness in every detail;	
Do you tend to believe that in general, there is only one right way to do things?		Believing that there is only one right way to do things;	
Do you often end up doing things yourself to make sure they are done right?			
Once you have formed an opinion about something, do you rarely change your mind because you know you're right?		Difficulty changing ideas and/or viewpoint;	
Are you the kind of person who focuses on details, order, and organization or who likes to make lists and schedules? Give me some examples.		Preoccupation with details, organization, and order.	

?	0	1	2	3
Insufficient information	Very little or not at all descriptive	Mildly descriptive	Moderately descriptive	Very descriptive

Disinhibition Domain Score

Record each <u>Disinhibition facet</u> score here:

Irresponsibility	_____
Impulsivity	_____
Distractibility	_____
Risk Taking	_____
The facet Rigid Perfectionism is not utilized in the domain score.	
Sum of the above scores (record on page 33, "Personality Trait Domain Profile")	_____
Average score (summed scores divided by 4) (record on page 33, "Summary of Average Domain Scores")	_____

?	0	1	2	3
Insufficient information	**Very little or not at all descriptive**	**Mildly descriptive**	**Moderately descriptive**	**Very descriptive**

PSYCHOTICISM DOMAIN

Exhibiting a wide range of culturally incongruent odd, eccentric, or unusual behaviors and cognitions, including both process (e.g., perception, dissociation) and content (e.g., beliefs).

Interview questions	Facets	General definition	Trait ratings
NOTE: FOR ANY "YES" ANSWER, OBTAIN DETAILS BEFORE MAKING THE RATING.	**Unusual Beliefs and Experiences** (an aspect of Psychoticism)		? 0 1 2 3
Do you sometimes believe that you can read other people's minds?		Belief that one has unusual abilities, such as mind reading, telekinesis, thought-action fusion;	
How about being able to physically move things simply by thinking about moving them?			
Have you sometimes felt that you could make things happen or influence people just by making a wish or thinking about them?			
Do you believe that you have a "sixth sense" that allows you to know and predict things that others can't?			
Have you had personal experiences with the supernatural?			
	(continued on next page)		

?	0	1	2	3
Insufficient information	Very little or not at all descriptive	Mildly descriptive	Moderately descriptive	Very descriptive

Interview questions	Facets	General definition	Trait ratings
	Unusual Beliefs and Experiences (*continued*)		
Have you had weird experiences that are difficult to explain?		Unusual experiences of reality, including hallucination-like experiences.	
Do you sometimes hear things that others can't hear?			
Do you see things that aren't actually there?			
Have you sometimes had the sense that some person or force is around you even though you cannot see anyone?			
Have you had any other experiences that you or someone else might consider unusual?			
ALSO CONSIDER INTERVIEWEE'S APPEARANCE AND BEHAVIOR DURING THE INTERVIEW.	**Eccentricity** (an aspect of Psychoticism)	Odd, unusual, or bizarre behavior, appearance, and/or speech;	**? 0 1 2 3**
Do you sometimes have the feeling that your thoughts are unpredictable?		Having strange and unpredictable thoughts;	
Do your thoughts often go off in odd or unusual directions?			
IF NO: **Have others told you that your thoughts do not make sense to them?**			
	(*continued on next page*)		

?	0	1	2	3
Insufficient information	Very little or not at all descriptive	Mildly descriptive	Moderately descriptive	Very descriptive

Interview questions	Facets	General definition	Trait ratings
Eccentricity (*continued*)			
Do other people seem to think your behavior is odd, eccentric, or weird?		Saying unusual or inappropriate things.	
Do others seem to think that you act, talk, or look odd, strange, or unusual?			
Have you been told that you have a number of odd quirks or habits?			
CONSIDER INTERVIEWEE'S SPEECH AND THINKING PROCESSES DURING THE INTERVIEW.	**Cognitive and Perceptual Dysregulation** (an aspect of Psychoticism)		? 0 1 2 3
Do your thoughts often go off in odd or unusual directions?		Odd or unusual thought processes and experiences, including depersonalization, derealization, and dissociative experiences;	
IF NO: Have others told you that your thoughts do not make sense to them?			
Do other people sometimes complain that when you speak, you veer off on tangents and have trouble getting to the point?			
Do other people often tell you that you are too vague when expressing yourself?			
Do other people often tell you that you go into too much detail when recounting a story?			
	(*continued on next page*)		

?	0	1	2	3
Insufficient information	Very little or not at all descriptive	Mildly descriptive	Moderately descriptive	Very descriptive

Interview questions	Facets	General definition	Trait ratings
	Cognitive and Perceptual Dysregulation (*continued*)		
Do you often have the feeling that everything is unreal or that you are in a dream, detached from your body or mind?			
What about feeling like you were an outside observer of your own thoughts or movements?			
Do you often "zone out" and then suddenly come to and realize that a lot of time has passed?			
Do people often talk about you doing things that you don't remember at all?			
Have you been having problems with your memory in general? Tell me about that.			
IF YES: **Were you drinking or taking drugs at the time?**			
Do you sometimes have trouble telling the difference between dreams and waking life?		Mixed sleep-wake state experiences;	
Do you sometimes feel as if an outside force or person is controlling what you think?		Thought-control experiences.	

?	0	1	2	3
Insufficient information	Very little or not at all descriptive	Mildly descriptive	Moderately descriptive	Very descriptive

Psychoticism Domain Score

Record each <u>Psychoticism facet</u> score here:

Unusual Beliefs and Experiences	_____
Eccentricity	_____
Cognitive and Perceptual Dysregulation	_____
Sum of the above scores (record on page 33, "Personality Trait Domain Profile")	_____
Average score (summed scores divided by 3) (record on page 33, "Summary of Average Domain Scores")	_____

?	0	1	2	3
Insufficient information	**Very little or not at all descriptive**	**Mildly descriptive**	**Moderately descriptive**	**Very descriptive**

PERSONALITY TRAIT DOMAIN PROFILE

Circle the TOTAL SUMMED SCORE for each domain.

Next, connect the circled scores with a line to create the profile:

Negative Affectivity (page 11)	0 1 2 3 4 5 6 7 8 9 10 11 12 13 14 15 16 17 18 19 20 21 22 23 24
Detachment (page 17)	0 1 2 3 4 5 6 7 8 9 10 11 12 13 14 15 16 17 18
Antagonism (page 22)	0 1 2 3 4 5 6 7 8 9 10 11 12 13 14 15 16 17 18
Disinhibition (page 27)	0 1 2 3 4 5 6 7 8 9 10 11 12
Psychoticism (page 32)	0 1 2 3 4 5 6 7 8 9

SUMMARY OF <u>AVERAGE</u> DOMAIN SCORES

Negative Affectivity Domain (page 11)	_____
Detachment Domain (page 17)	_____
Antagonism Domain (page 22)	_____
Disinhibition Domain (page 27)	_____
Psychoticism Domain (page 32)	_____

EXPERTLY DESIGNED, the *Structured Clinical Interview for the DSM-5® Alternative Model for Personality Disorders* (SCID-5-AMPD) is a semi-structured diagnostic interview that guides clear assessment of the defining components of personality pathology as presented in the DSM-5 Alternative Model. The modular format of the SCID-5-AMPD allows the researcher or clinician to focus on those aspects of the Alternative Model of most interest.

Module II: Structured Clinical Interview for Personality Traits focuses on the dimensional assessment of the five pathological personality trait domains in the Alternative Model and their corresponding 25 trait facets. This comprehensive review of the trait domains (Negative Affectivity, Detachment, Antagonism, Disinhibition, and Psychoticism) identifies multiple areas of personality variation and provides a visual profile of scores across the trait domains.

Module II can be used independently or in combination with any of the following SCID-5-AMPD modules:

- **Module I** dimensionally assesses self and interpersonal functioning using the Level of Personality Functioning Scale.
- **Module III** comprehensively assesses each of the six specific personality disorders of the Alternative Model, as well as Personality Disorder–Trait Specified.

Also available is the **User's Guide for the SCID-5-AMPD:** the essential tool for the effective use of each SCID-5-AMPD module. This companion guide provides instructions for each SCID-5-AMPD module and features completed samples of all modules in full, with corresponding sample patient cases and commentary.

Trained clinicians with a basic knowledge of the concepts of personality and personality psychopathology will benefit from the myriad applications and perspectives offered by the SCID-5-AMPD.

ANDREW E. SKODOL, M.D., is Research Professor of Psychiatry at the University of Arizona College of Medicine in Tucson, Arizona, and Adjunct Professor of Psychiatry at Columbia University College of Physicians and Surgeons in New York, New York.

MICHAEL B. FIRST, M.D., is Professor of Clinical Psychiatry at Columbia University College of Physicians and Surgeons, and Research Psychiatrist in the Division of Clinical Phenomenology at the New York State Psychiatric Institute in New York, New York.

DONNA S. BENDER, PH.D., is Director, Counseling and Psychological Services, and Clinical Professor of Psychiatry and Behavioral Sciences at Tulane University in New Orleans, Louisiana.

JOHN M. OLDHAM, M.D., is Professor of Psychiatry and Barbara and Corbin Robertson Jr. Endowed Chair for Personality Disorders at Baylor College of Medicine in Houston, Texas.

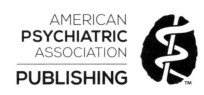

AMERICAN
PSYCHIATRIC
ASSOCIATION
PUBLISHING

WWW.APPI.ORG